Clergy

Physical

Health

____

Clergy Physical Health

Volume 4 of HCMHC

Stephen McCutchan

www.smccutchan.com

Clergy Physical Health/ Stephen McCutchan. -- 1st ed.

ISBN: 9781983181689

Dedicated to

Dr. Samuel Stevenson

My friend and colleague in ministry

And to

All the courageous clergy

Who have responded to God's call to ministry

Join my email list, ask for a free pdf on clergy care, and see all my

resources at stephenmccutchan@gmail.com

"... your body is a temple of the Holy Spirit within

you, which you have from God, ...

you are not your own"

–1 Corinthians 6:19

This book is a resource for clergy, congregations, and regional committees responsible for the care of clergy.

- Clergy can evaluate their own health and take specific steps to maintain or improve their health.
- Congregations can develop a strategy to nurture the health of their staff.
- Regional bodies can engage congregations and clergy in conversations and actions that promote healthier clergy and congregations.
-

God's call to ministry is both satisfying and challenging. This book offers practical ways to engage in ministry in a healthy manner.
If you are clergy, have a friend who is clergy, or want your congregation to be healthy, read, and act on the suggestions. Share it with others who care about the church and want to be inspired by the very best.

TABLE OF CONTENTS

HEALTHY CLERGY

MAKE

HEALTHY

CONGREGATIONS

An Overview

Like most of the biblical figures, clergy are not perfect, but God has an amazing way of working through those God has called to speak grace to the world.

The following pages are meant to provide you optional strategies that can nurture your health as well as stimulating your imagination to discover a variety of alternatives.

Some Disturbing statistics

If you have ever wondered why we should spend so much energy on how to care for clergy, take a look at some of these disturbing statistics on Parish Clergy Stress.

Lutheran Church–Missouri Synod Study

20% burned out

20% in advanced stages of burnout

When asked, "What is it like being a parish pastor these days?" two-thirds of the responses were negative:

-church conflict—people beating on each other

-mismatch of pastors and congregations

-the difficulty of getting help to pastors

-poor support for clergy spouses and children

-low clergy income

-grossly unreasonable expectations of the pastor

-infighting, dysfunctional congregations

-congregations where a few members dominate the whole leadership of the church

Fuller Institute of Church Growth

Surveyed 1,000 pastors:

-80% believe pastoral ministry has negatively affected their families

-75% reported a significant stress-related crisis at least once in their ministry

-50% felt unable to meet demands of the job

-90% felt inadequately trained to cope with ministry demands

-70% have a lower self-image than when they began their profession

-50% had considered leaving the ministry within three months prior to the survey

Mark Driscoll 2006 Study:

-1500 pastors per month leave ministry due to spiritual burnout, contention, or moral failures

-80% of pastors and 84% of spouses feel unqualified and discouraged in their role as pastors

-50% of pastors are so discouraged they would leave the ministry if could make another living

-80% of seminary and Bible school graduates who enter the ministry will leave within five years.

SIX ASPECTS OF

HEALTHY CLERGY

In this book, we will focus on physical health. In future volumes, we will look at emotional health, family health, financial health, spiritual health, and vocational health. All of us could be healthier in all six areas, and we will explore specific strategies by which we can contribute to improving our health.

Each aspect of health affects the other aspects. If you are emotionally stressed, it affects you physically. It can affect your family relationships, your sense of vocation, etc.

A person's health is not just an individual challenge. It is affected by our environment, our relationships, etc. So as we examine each of these areas, we will look at them not only from the perspective of the individual clergy/religious leader but also how they can be affected by both the congregation and the presbytery or judicatory.

If you are in a nonparish form of ministry or serve a church as an educator, musician, administrator, etc. challenges are the same, but some of the vocabularies may need to be adjusted.

If you would like to be informed of the publication of future books in the series and informed of future developments in the search for healthy congregations and healthy clergy, you are invited to sign up at www.smccutchan.com.

Direct your questions and suggestions to steve@smccutchan.com.

CLERGY

DON'T HAVE IT ALL TOGETHER

Clergy, like all humans, come to their work with all the wounds, hungers, insecurities, and troubles of their past. As the Bible makes clear, being called by God does not perfect the person. As our seminaries demonstrate, you do not perfect a person through education. We are the imperfect servants of God through whom God chooses to work to achieve the divine purpose.

So when I say Healthy Clergy Make Healthy Congregations, I recognize that we are at best speaking of "Wounded Healers." However, a vital issue for clergy is whether they can respond to the unhealthy dynamics they encounter in a congregation and in ministry in a healthy manner.

IMPERFECT CLERGY MAKE HEALTHY RESPONSES

Consider some of the healthy responses that clergy can make in a congregation. As you read each of them, give yourself a rating 1-5, five being the most like your response. Be as honest as you can.

1. By faith, they believe they are worthy but not perfect. They are willing to learn from their mistakes.

2. They are not afraid to acknowledge their own weaknesses, doubts, and concerns but do not let them become a narcissistic focus of their ministry. They recognize that many of the issues that arise are not a reflection of their worthiness.

3. They do not ask perfection of themselves or members of the congregation. They are not afraid to fail.

4. They believe that their congregation, with all its strengths and weaknesses, is sufficient to be the Body of Christ, and therefore they explore their issues and challenges as an opportunity to grow in faith.

5. They dare to embrace the vulnerability of their life together with compassion for all involved, believing that with risk comes creativity, courage, innovation, and growth in faith.

6. They are willing to help the congregation surface any shame in their history that binds them and demonstrate the empathy that is an antidote to the shame.

7. They demonstrate practices of gratitude and joy.

Consider evaluating yourself. Be as honest as you can.

EMBRACING THE CHRIST WITHIN US

Healthy clergy know:

(Rate yourself from 1-5)

- They don't have all the answers

- That the best of plans can fail

- That the demonic is expressed in silence, secrecy, and judgment of each other.

Healthy clergy seek:

- To exegete the word of God incarnated in the Body of Christ

- To trust that sin does not defeat God

- To seek God's purpose even in the worst of circumstances.

Healthy clergy recognize:

- They are called to serve God rather than the reverse
- Not all service is going to be comfortable.

How have you rated yourself? What would you add or change to the characteristics of healthy clergy? To be healthy is more than just physical health, but it certainly includes our physical health.

STEWARDSHIP

OF

SELF

PHYSICAL CARE OF SELF IN MINISTRY

In one sense it is obvious, but there is evidence that clergy do not take care of themselves physically. We are engaged in a stressful profession and neglecting our bodies makes us very vulnerable. Everyone knows that in the abstract, but it is easy to overlook the care of our bodies in practice.

The most obvious areas of care for our bodies are diet and physical exercise.

Begin with becoming conscious of your reality. Take a piece of paper and list some ways you are currently paying attention to your diet and getting your exercise. Are you pleased with the result? While you are at it, identify a first step in improving your behavior.

An ethics book I read described the temptation of small indulgences. For example, I might say, "I've been working hard, doing so much good, I deserve that candy bar or extra order of french fries." OR "I've been so busy meeting the demands of my congregation that I have just been too tired to go exercise." On your paper, list a couple of small indulgences that you have given in to during the past month.

Not all indulgences are wrong, but they can quickly get out of hand. Becoming conscious of them is a first step to keeping a balance in your life.

Don't set yourself up for failure by comparing what you do now with some ideal that is impossible to achieve. Think about one small step you can take and let that be a beginning. Also identify the type of social support that you need to make this small step.

Your Body Is a Temple

We are going through a difficult time for clergy. There is clear evidence that the stress and demands of ministry are having a significant adverse effect on the physical health of clergy. Even if you think that you are not one of those who has poor health, it is important to occasionally stop and ask yourself how you are doing physically and whether you need to alter some practices that might be hard on your health.

By virtue of our call, we are not our own. We have been set aside by God for a purpose. As part of our responding to that call, we need to pay attention to our physical wellbeing. Like all human beings, we are subject to the stresses of our culture. Therefore, we need to be intentional about caring for our physical selves.

First, make an appointment to have a good physical with a doctor at least once a year. It is not good stewardship of the body in which you were born to neglect this. Most denominations see this as so necessary that the medical plans have incentives for doing so. Even if you do not have good insurance, it is still cost-effective to get a yearly physical.

Second, when we are honest with ourselves, we can identify ways to improve our health. Take a piece of paper and write for ten minutes on your personal eating and snacking habits and how they do or do not contribute to your health. Then survey your sleep habits over the past month. How frequently is your sleep interrupted by other people, your work habits, and your feelings of stress and anxiety? Now, do the same with the exercise you are getting. One pastor bought a pedometer and strapped it on each day to note whether his day had been mostly sedentary or whether he had done some active walking. In addition to intentional exercise, we can often get some benefits by choosing to park in spots that allow us to walk further, taking stairs rather than elevators, etc.

A YMCA, YWCA, or sports club are familiar places for regular exercise. Many have trainers at reasonable rates. Having a trainer to whom you are accountable helps establish a good exercise routine.

Look at some of the ways people get exercise in connection with other people. Some play sports, attend exercise classes, find a partner to walk with, run with, etc. Who do you know who might enjoy partnering with you to begin a better exercise program? Having someone else who expects you to participate helps build support for changing your habits. I played racquetball early in the morning. Knowing that someone was on the courts waiting for me was a strong incentive to get out of bed and get going. Some people have found the same value in an early morning or evening walking partner. Your body is a temple of God. Use it in a way that brings praise.

Third, it is not unusual in our culture to respond to stress by eating or drinking in an unhealthy manner. As pastors and educators (P/E), we need to take seriously that this is a spiritual issue. As Paul reminds us in 1 Corinthians 6:19, "Do you not know that your body is a temple (or sanctuary) of the Holy Spirit within you, which you have from God, and that you are not your own? Take another piece of paper and describe how you are currently paying attention to your diet, sleep habits, and exercise. Are you pleased with the result? While you are at it, describe a first step in improving your behavior.

Self-Care As a Witness

A significant barrier to clergy taking care of themselves is the attitude of the clergy themselves. Most of us responded to the call to ministry assuming that there would be a measure of sacrifice to our service. Too much focus on self-care seems contradictory to the nobleness of our call. The majority of clergy are more comfortable giving than receiving care. It makes us nervous to be on the receiving end of too much personal attention.

Fourth, a somewhat scary step is to explore the spiritual dimensions of taking care of your physical body by preaching or teaching a course on it. Then share with your congregation your desire to improve your body and invite them to do the same. There is nothing like public commitment to strengthen your resolve. The management of time in a way that enables us to live a healthy life is a significant issue for our whole society. If clergy, who have a very demanding profession, can also demonstrate how to balance the demands of their ministry with their personal and social needs, it is a significant witness to a society that reveals an inability to manage time and experience life fully. The issue of balance between work, rest, and social relationships is one of the crucial areas of our society. While there are people, including clergy, who are very adept at caring for themselves, many in our community are unsuccessful in achieving a healthy balance.

One place to start is to probe the wisdom of the Sabbath commandment in the Judeo-Christian faith. It was an original contribution to the meaning of time and human behavior. You will note that this commandment has a more extended explanation than any of the other commandments. It also receives a different explanation in the Exodus list of commandments than in the list in Deuteronomy. It was as if writers of both books realized that this commandment would be harder to understand than the others, so it needed additional explanation.

As Jesus demonstrated, the issue is not adherence to some modern form of *blue laws.* Rather, it is the truth and wisdom of honoring the Sabbath. It sets up a balance and rhythm of work and rest. Both productivity and relationships with God and neighbor are critical for a fulfilling life. Engage colleagues and members of your congregation in exploring that wisdom.

EVALUATING

SELF

SELF-EVALUATION

As you review the list below, make a check mark beside the items that you regularly practice and an X beside those things that you would like to explore.

PHYSICAL HEALTH CHECKLIST

1. Yearly physical check-up.

2. An exercise program that you practice.

Does it have both a strength component and a cardio component?

3. A sport that you participate in that helps you stay in shape.

4. Evaluate your diet? Do you try to have a balanced diet and limit your intake of unhealthy foods?

5. Is your weight within a healthy margin? You can Google suggested healthy weights.

6. Do you belong to a Y or sports club that encourages you to exercise?

7. Do you have a home exercise machine?

8. Do you participate in yoga, tai chi, Pilate, or some other stretch and relax program?

9. Do you have a partner(s) that help you stay accountable for your exercising?

10. Are you part of either a running or walking regimen?

11. Do you have a mini-exercise routine that you can use when you are traveling or limited in time?

12. Do you know how to practice meditation or relaxation breathing when you are under stress?

13. Are you are aware of signs of stress in your body that alert you to the need to practice some relaxation techniques?

14. Are you are familiar with some basic first aid if you should experience injury?

15. Do you get sufficient sleep to restore your body?

16. Are you are aware of specific techniques to assist you when you have trouble sleeping?

Your physical health is vital. Choose the top eight in priority order for you. Ask a friend to do the same. Compare your lists and see if the conversation alters your priorities.

Another way to evaluate your approach to physical health is to make use of "A List of Ten."

A LIST OF TEN

Making a list of ten is a simple discipline that can offer surprising results. By making a list of ten, we push ourselves beyond the surface reflections and begin to delve beneath the surface. Apply this discipline to your physical health. It's simple to do and can be very revealing to you.

List the ten ways that a pastor can maintain his or her physical health while responding to the demands of the ministry. I phrase it that way because I think we always need to keep the perspective of being called by God to this ministry even as we seek to take care of ourselves.

When I begin to make a list of ten ways to take care of myself physically, the first few are easy to list even if I don't always follow them.

1. I can get some regular good physical exercise.

2. I can eat well-balanced meals and avoid junk food.

3. I can strive to get sufficient sleep.

4. That one is not as easy as it first seems. Doctors say we should average eight hours of sleep a night. I rarely did that during my forty years of ministry. At the same time, I did try to pay attention to getting an average of six and occasionally increased it to eight.

5. I can receive regular physical checkups and listen to what the doctor tells me.

6. I can find a fun hobby that involves some physical exertion which combines fun and physical exercise.

7. I can recognize the importance of having a few good relationships that nurture me. In my case that begins with my wife, but for others it may mean some good friends that you regularly meet with for conversation.

8. I can pay attention to my emotional thermometer and be honest with myself about how I am feeling at various moments in my life. These last two begin to merge into paying attention to my emotional health, but they also affect my physical health.

OK, it's your turn. Either take out a piece of paper or bring up a new screen on your computer/notebook. Do not look back at my items until you have identified ten ways. Do not worry about how realistic your ideas are until you have allowed yourself to complete your list. There will be plenty of time to edit your suggestions later.

Perhaps you should take a deeper look at your choices.

TAKING A DEEPER LOOK

Using the same discipline of a list of ten, extend your reflections and learn something new about yourself by making a second list of ten. This time, make a list of ten statements about the excuses you can use to avoid taking better care of yourself physically.

1. One excuse I use is . . .

2. Another excuse is . . .

3. I also . . .

DON'T STOP NOW.

The more you are aware of your excuses, the more control you have over your own behavior.

STEPS TO

PHYSICAL

HEALTH

CONSIDER THE PRICE WE PAY

When your physical health declines, the social, emotional, and spiritual challenges of ministry can escalate. A physical exercise program can reduce the risk of diabetes, heart disease, and cancer. Drawing on information I found at, http://www.journeyworks.com, Journeyworks Publishing, I want to share some ideas on how to improve your physical health.

Experts say that 30 to 60 minutes of physical activity on most days can improve your health significantly. While many busy people have difficulty finding 60 minutes to set aside for exercise, what you may not know is that you can break up that 30 to 60 minutes into bite-size chunks and still get the benefits. According to a Journeyworks brochure, if you can find blocks of ten minutes and engage in activity that makes your heart beat faster, you can benefit.

Let me offer twenty-one ideas to spark your imagination. Of course, none of them will work unless you do them. The important thing is to become intentional about achieving some exercise throughout your week. As you look at these ideas, and others that may come to you, also think about your week and where you can plug them in. By putting exercise on your calendar, you will be more likely to engage in some activity. Otherwise, you might have good intentions but come to the end of the week and realize that you have forgotten.

Make a game out of it by giving yourself points every time you exercise and plan a reward when you have reached your chosen score. Just make sure that the prize is healthy as well.

TWENTY-ONE SUGGESTIONS

1. Think of housecleaning as an opportunity to do some bending and stretching.

2. Skip the elevator during hospital visits and choose the stairs.

3. Instead of meeting a friend for lunch, suggest meeting and talking with your friend while you are walking.

4. Instead of driving around seeking the closest parking space, deliberately choose one that is further away and do a little walking. However, do remember where you parked, or you may do a lot of walking.

5. Instead of a riding mower, choose a push mower, and a snow shovel instead of a snowplow. Both of these activities can get your heart beating pretty quickly. Do be careful as you begin not to overdo it.

6.   Be considerate of your neighbors and choose to rake your leaves instead of picking the noisiest leaf blower in the neighborhood.

7.   Walk or ride a bike to work or when you are visiting members. You will be preaching a sermon on the environment while you improve your health.

8.   Group your errands so that you can include some extra walking while you are shopping. Sometimes shopping can be beneficial if you don't succumb to the temptation to reward yourself with a high-calorie drink.

9.   Instead of being a couch potato in front of the TV, make use of an exercise machine while you are watching your favorite program. It's a great way to ease the guilt of workaholics while you are still enjoying your program.

10.   Make a regular appointment with a friend to play tennis, basketball, etc. When someone else is

expecting you, you are not as likely to find an excuse not to go.

11. There are some great workout videos, yoga videos, or others that you can use in the privacy of your home. Of course, if a family member can be encouraged to join you, then there is some valuable bonding that can take place at the same time.

12. Dance classes, aerobic classes, spinning classes, and many other opportunities await the person who looks for them.

13. Choose a sport that you enjoy and look for a team in your community that you can join. Participation is a lot better for you than being a spectator.

14. Walking a pet can contribute to your health. Choose a pet that will push you a little on your walk. Find a friend who also has a pet and plan some joint walks.

15. Choose activities on your day off that engage you physically. Maybe visit a park with walking trails. If you have children, try flying a kite or playing catch.

16. Find some rhythmic music that you enjoy and find a private place where you can overcome your inhibitions and dance with lots of body movement.

17. Build in some stretching and jogging to your morning wake up routine. You don't have to be a marathon runner to gain the benefit.

18. Bike riding, especially with members of your family, can have multiple benefits.

19. Be charitable while taking care of yourself by joining in the fund-raising walks and runs. It is not who comes in first, and its lots of fun.

20. Invite some members of your congregation to go bowling, skating, hiking, etc. You build community among your congregants while you are contributing to both their health and yours.

21. Make it a congregation wide project to discover many little ways that the members can get exercise and award points for activities so that it is a fun, public way to improve everyone's health. Consider it

another angle on the stewardship of the body that God has provided us.

Many times, problems in the ministry can be converted to possibilities if you reframe them. We can make the noblest of excuses for our failure to take care of our health because we are too busy taking care of others. However, the problem of declining physical health is not restricted to pastors but is rampant in our society.

SO HERE IS THE CHALLENGE:

Pick out two or three of the most interesting suggestions and act on them. Keeping the body healthy within the Body of Christ is one facet of living out our faith.

60 SECOND EXERCISES

I found a Website that is focused on physical health and offers a set of 60-second aerobics that you can do in the office. More information is available for you at the

Website, www.webmd.com An article by Jean Lawrence on exercises you can do at your desk is one among many of their valuable articles. Here is a peek at some of what they offer:

60 SECOND AEROBICS

To improve your heart rate variability—your heart's ability to jump from resting to "pumped"—has been shown to increase longevity and decrease heart disease risk.

While you should not give up on your home or gym exercise routine, you can certainly supplement it with exercises done at your desk (and, on those extra-long workdays, it's much better than doing nothing.) Here are a few aerobic tricks to try during your next break between tasks:

Glance at the wall clock and rip off a minute's worth of jumping jacks. If you're a beginner, try the low-impact version (raise your right arm and tap your left toe to the side while keeping your right foot on the floor; alternate sides).

Do a football-like drill of running in place for 60 seconds. Get those knees up! (Beginners, march in place.)

Simulate jumping rope for a minute: Hop on alternate feet, or on both feet at once. A more relaxed version is to simulate the arm motion of turning a rope, while alternately tapping the toes of each leg in front.

While seated, pump both arms over your head for 30 seconds and then rapidly tap your feet on the floor, football-drill style, for 30 seconds. Repeat 3-5 times.

If you can step into a vacant office or conference room, shadow box for a minute or two. Or just walk around the room as fast as you can.

Or do walk-lunges in your office or a vacant room. (You could also amuse your coworkers by doing these in the hall; remember Monty Python's "Ministry of Silly Walks" comedy routine?). Set your PDA to beep you into action.

No conference room? Take to the stairs —two at a time if you need a harder workout! Do this 5-7 times a day.

Some strength-building suggestions:

Do one-legged squats (hold onto a wall or table for support) while waiting for a Website page to load, the copier to spit our your reports, or faxes to slither out.

Stand with one leg straight and try to kick your buttocks with the other.

Sitting in your chair, lift one leg off the seat, extend it out straight, hold for 2 seconds; then lower your foot (stop short of the floor) and hold for several seconds. Switch; do each leg 15 times.

To work your chest and shoulders, place both hands on your chair arms and slowly lift your bottom off the chair. Lower yourself back down, but stop short of the seat, hold for a few seconds. Do 15 times.

To stretch your back and strengthen your biceps, place your hands on the desk and hang on. Slowly push your chair back until your head is between your arms, and you're looking at the floor. Then slowly pull yourself back in. Again, do 15 of these.

Desk push-ups can be a good strengthener. (First, make sure your desk is stable enough to support your weight.) Standing, put your hands on the desk. Walk backward, then do push-ups against the desk. Repeat 15 times.

Reach for the Sky

Stretching exercises are a natural for the desk-bound, to ease stress and keep your muscles from clenching up. Here are a few suggestions:

Sitting tall in your chair, stretch both arms over your head and reach for the sky. After 10 seconds, extend the right hand higher, then the left.

Let your head loll over so that your right ear nearly touches your right shoulder. Using your hand, press your head a little lower (gently, now). Hold for 10 seconds. Relax, and then repeat on the other side.

Try this yoga posture to relieve tension: Sit facing forward, then turn your head to the left and your torso to the right and hold a few seconds. Repeat 15 times, alternating sides.

Sitting up straight, try to touch your shoulder blades together. Hold, and then relax.

You get to put your feet up for this one! To ease the hamstrings and lower back, push your chair away from your desk, and put your right heel up on the desk. Sit up straight, and bend forward just until you feel a gentle stretch in the back of your leg. Flex your foot for a few seconds, and then point it. Lean forward a little farther, flex your foot again, and hold for 10 seconds. Repeat on the other side.

Unobtrusive But Effective

Women can do Kegels—tightening and holding, then loosening, their pelvic floor muscles (the muscles that control the flow of urine when you go to the bathroom). This will prevent leakage and other problems down the line.

Butt clenches are also helpful in today's booty-conscious society. Tighten your buttocks, hold, hold, hold, and then relax. Repeat 15 times. The same goes for ab squeezes—just tighten your tummy muscles instead.

One last thing: Do not let fear of embarrassment keep you from exercising at work. Chances are, your co-workers will admire your efforts rather than be amused. You might even get them to join you for a lunchtime walk or to help you lobby for lunch-hour yoga classes at your workplace.

There is more on their Website. It might be a way to begin or continue taking care of your physical body during a busy profession.

FAITHFUL

EATING

THE RISING WEIGHT OF CLERGY

In 2009 Presbyterians Today reported in their March issue a startling study of the changing weight of pastors. In 17 years the average weight of pastors increased 11 pounds, from 181 pounds in 1991 to 192 pounds in 2008. The share of pastors who are obese doubled from 14 percent to 27 percent in that time period. This increase, according to their study, occurred for both male and female pastors, and younger and older pastors. This is not the type of equality that we are seeking.

I am assuming that this is happening in other denominations as well. This increase in obesity follows the national trend towards obesity among the general populace. There is evidence that this tendency towards obesity affects clergy's mental health. Is it possible that it also affects their spiritual health and their capacity to engage in productive ministry?

I realize that there is a built-in prejudice against heavy people. There is no physical description of Jesus in the Scriptures. Our images have been developed out of our imagination. Still, have you ever seen a picture of a fat Jesus or even a heavy-set Jesus? Contrast that to the Asian image of a fat Buddha.

There is a good reason to examine our prejudice regarding weight, but we also need to recognize the health costs, both mentally and physically, of inappropriate weight. And we should ask what this increase in obesity among our clergy is saying about how they handle the stress and challenges of ministry.

On the positive side, the same report found that 21 percent of Presbyterian clergy are in formal weight-loss programs and 39 percent belong to fitness centers. The complete survey is at www.pcusa.olrg/research.

SEVEN SMALL STEPS

TO A HEALTHIER YOU

Let me suggest some simple steps that you can take over a series of months.

It all begins by our deciding to take the first step and then deciding on the next step. Feel free to be innovative and creative in your approach. Rather than make it one more burden in an already overtaxed life, try to make it more like a game.

The **FIRST STEP** is to raise the issue of food out of a routine unconscious practice and to become intentional about what you eat. Many years ago, I read about a strategy by Smoke-Enders that was used to build awareness for people who wanted to stop smoking. The first step, they suggested, was to stick a small card in a packet of cigarettes and date the time and place when they had a cigarette. The idea was to make one aware of what had often become an unconscious habit. So, for you, buy a small pocket calendar or notepad and make a note each time you have something to drink or eat and what it was.

STEP TWO would be to Google healthy and unhealthy foods and make a list of ten healthy and ten unhealthy foods that you like to eat. Make the list of ten foods that are frequently part of your eating pattern. It's cheating to list alligator meat as one of the unhealthy foods you want to avoid.

Now with your list in mind, keep track of your eating habits for a month and give yourself a score of plus 5 for each healthy food you eat and minus 5 for each unhealthy food. Even if the food is not on your list, you might want to give it a score. Make a note at the end of each week of whether you are in the positive or negative scoring area.

STEP THREE is to focus your attention on consuming fruits and vegetables. Depending on your size and age, healthy living suggests you eat between 5 and 13 servings of fruits and vegetables a day. In your case, make note of how many servings you now eat. The Website for *Cooking Light* has some instructions on how to measure servings and a downloadable calendar for keeping track. A beginning would be to intentionally add one extra serving for at least two meals a day. It can be as simple as eating an extra banana or apple as a snack food.

STEP FOUR would be to become conscious of how frequently you make use of having a snack or drink not because you are hungry but because you need a break. Have some fun with a colleague by brainstorming a variety of 10 to 15-minute break ideas that would be enjoyable but not add to your calorie intake. Many people used to smoke a cigarette for that break. That's not a good idea, but you can be creative in choosing more healthy alternatives. Because you are opting out of eating, it might be a good idea to begin with something that involves your lips and your hands. A glass of ice water might substitute for a Coke.

STEP FIVE as a clergy person is to consider the spiritual and theological implications of what you are trying to do. You might do some research on the ways food plays a role in the practice of faith and build a sermon around what you learn. There is a reason why fasting is significant in the faith story. It is not an accident that food and drink were the common elements used in the central acts of worship for both Jews and Christians.

STEP SIX might encourage other members of your congregation or other clergy friends to join you in building support for a healthier diet. Each of you might do some research in a particular area of eating healthy and share your findings. It is a solid principle that making use of both the support of and accountability to others in making changes can increase your success rate.

STEP SEVEN might be to build a list of what you think are the most weight-producing foods you eat over a month's time. The first step is not to stop eating them but just to notice what you do eat. Once you become more aware, do some research on what might be some pleasurable but healthier substitutes. At some point in this process, you might want to note which of your changes are having a positive impact on your weight.

There are many programs like Weight Watchers, or others, that can be helpful. What I have tried to do is to suggest possibilities that do not require a lot of additional time commitments as a way of integrating new habits into your busy life.

EATING YOUR WAY TO HAPPINESS

You have read the articles pointing out the rise in obesity among the clergy. You recognize the tendency to think "ain't it awful" about those other grossly overweight clergy. You may have excused yourself as a naturally large person or even thought to yourself "Someday I should really focus on reducing my weight." Consider that the issue of healthy eating is not separate from your practice of ministry but can be an integral part of your ministry.

FIVE UNCOMFORTABLE QUESTIONS

1. Is it possible that you would improve your chance for longevity if you intentionally lost some weight and kept it off?

2. Is it possible that your poor eating habits and weight gain do reflect some unresolved emotional issues in your life?

3. Is it possible that keeping yourself in a healthy state has some spiritual implications?

4. Are there some spiritual truths embedded in the many places in Scripture where food becomes part of the conversation?

5. Are there ways that eating correctly can be a spiritual witness that can touch others?

Or, to summarize, can you as a pastor pay attention to what you eat as part of your healing message to your congregation and your colleagues?

THE TRUTH IS

Dan Buettner, in his book Blue Zones Solution, reports on his study of groups of people around the world who tend to live longer than others. One of his conclusions, which is supported by many other studies as well as common sense, is that what we eat significantly affects how long we will live. Buettner reports that the world's most robust 100 year-olds stick with diets that are 95% plant-based. The University of Southern California's Longevity Institute studies show that people with the highest protein intake have the highest risk of cancer and cardiovascular diseases. Protein from animals activates two sets of genes that accelerate aging. Most of us vaguely know this but indulge in foods that cumulatively threaten our health

If we were counseling someone else, we could point out all the forms of denial and rationalizations people use. Perhaps a major one is most of us live in denial of our death. It is not only teenagers but many of us who live as if we were immortal. Yet, as Christians, we have a faith that invites us to be good stewards of what God has given us, including our bodies. The health crisis among the clergy does raise some significant spiritual issues.

Wisdom suggests that we do not confront significant issues by seeking one big solution. Nor do we make much progress by guilt. We begin where we are and take small steps that are easily within our control. Success builds on success and encourages us to continue in a positive direction.

Family Obesity

Clergy families have not escaped the challenge of obesity that is plaguing our nation. Some denominational studies suggest that pastors may be even more challenged by the problem of obesity than the average population. If this is a problem in your family, you may want to address it as a total family and draw upon the spiritual resources that are available to you. I will suggest a procedure that assumes that the children are old enough to write. Adjustments will need to be made for younger children.

First have a family discussion around 1 Corinthians 3:16-17. "Do you not know that you are God's temple and that God's Spirit dwells in you? If anyone destroys God's temple, God will destroy that person. For God's temple is holy, and you are that temple." Let everyone express their opinion about what they hear in that passage that speaks to the problem of obesity in their family.

When you are finished, let each person write down

two or three things s/he personally does that

contributes to the weight problem and

one or two things that a person might do that would

begin to address that issue.

When all have shared, recognize that the problem

is not easy to change and let each person name

one first step that a person might take and

support that person needs from the other members

of the family.

After each person has shared, then discuss

covenanting together to help each other. It is helpful to

begin with small steps and build in ways to check in with

each other on a regular basis. Also, discuss how to

respond as a family when any member fails to complete

their objective so that the person can begin again. Do not

build on guilt but instead on support and affirmation.

Complete the covenanting with a family prayer. We all need to support each other. That's what healthy families do.

Changing Eating Habits

The following is taken from the newsletter of the ECLA Board of Pensions' Website, https://www.porticobenefits.org, which has excellent suggestions in a variety of ways to nurture your health. This one is focused on our physical health. www.elcabop.org

Tackle a Habit

(The Mayo Clinic Diet, 2010)

Week One– Consider five food-related habits.

1. **Skipping breakfast**, "*I skip breakfast.*"

For one week, eat a healthy breakfast every morning. It does not have to be a whole meal. If you want, start with a piece of fruit. Why tackle this habit? Evidence suggests people who eat breakfast manage their weight better than those who skip breakfast. Their performance during the day tends to be better, and they are less likely to feel ravenous and overeat later in the day.

2. **Snacks**, "I reach for unhealthy snacks."

For one week, if you want a snack, reach for a healthy snack—fruit, vegetable, whole grains or nuts. No other snacks allowed. Why tackle this habit? The typical salty or sweet processed snacks have lots of calories and little food value. Vegetables and fruits have just the opposite—few calories and lots of food value. They're nutritious and will fill you up without loading you up with calories.

3. **Indulging a sweet tooth**, "I can't resist a candy bar at the checkout counter."

For one week, if you want something sweet, eat fresh fruit. Eat no sugar from familiar sources: candy, table sugar, brown sugar, honey, jam, jelly, desserts, or sodas. Why tackle this habit? Sugar has calories but no nutritional value. Yet it is an increasing part of the American diet and a contributor to the increase in obesity.

4. **Loading up on meat,** "I make meat the star of my meals."

For one week, limit your servings of meat, poultry, and fish to 3 ounces (the size of a standard deck of cards). Give the starring role on your plate to vegetables and fruits. Why tackle this habit? Even lean cuts of meat and skinless poultry have some saturated fat and cholesterol and can be high in calories. And many non-meat low-calorie alternatives offer protein. See

https://www.nomeatathlete.com/vegetarian-protein/

as one list of suggestions.

5. I avoid whole grains,"I choose white bread and rice."

For one week, buy and eat only whole-grain bread, pasta, brown rice, and oatmeal. Why tackle this habit? Whole grain products are made with the entire grain kernel which is filled with vitamins, minerals, and fiber. They add bulk, help fill you up and reduce your risk of being overweight.

MAKE A CHOICE

Choose the habit you're . . . um . . . familiar with.

Starting with the Mayo Clinic link provided below, read up on information related to the habit you want to break. Purchase foods (if appropriate) to help you make better choices. Then, pick your start date, and steel your resolve to tackle your habit for just one week.

During the week, notice what's hard, what's not, what supported you, what didn't. How would you continue beyond your week? Take notes on your calendar.

Next three weeks–If you choose to, continue for three more weeks, but in a more relaxed way. For example, let's say you tackle the habit, "I indulge my sweet tooth." For week one, you avoided sugar completely. Now, occasionally, allow yourself a sugary dessert. Most of the time, however, choose fresh fruit.

During these three weeks, notice what helps you stay on track. Recognize when it pays to ease up. Continue tracking your progress on your calendar.

Go to the Mayo Website *https://www.mayoclinic.org/healthy-lifestyle/weight-loss/in-depth/mayo-clinic-diet/art-20045460* and see some helpful links to develop these themes further.

STRESS

AND

HEALTH

Remembering to Breathe

The following is taken from the excellent newsletter of the Laurence Schmidt Center _www.veralloyd.org,_ which is worth subscribing to.

Calm Your Nerves with Relaxation Exercises

By Madeline Vann, MPH

Breathing exercises are the mainstay of relaxation exercises that you can do anywhere at any time. And they can make a world of difference in how you feel.

Try it: Take a deep, slow breath and exhale—and repeat the process one more time. Do you feel better?

When we are stressed, our muscles tighten up, and our breathing changes and becomes shallow. As you breathe more lightly, you are participating in a vicious circle because your body responds to the change in breathing with a fight-or-flight response, adding to your tension and stress.

The most basic thing you can do when you start to feel stressed out is to stop and take some deep, even, slow breaths.

"If you sit and even just take five or ten deep breaths and try to relax your breathing, that can be tremendously helpful," says Mary Coussons-Read, Ph.D., professor of psychology, health and behavioral sciences and associate dean of the University of Colorado in Denver.

Sometimes it is remembering the little things that we can do when we are tense that can make a significant difference.

In that same article, Mary Coussons-Read, Ph.D., suggests some additional small tricks to enhance relaxation.

Try Visualization

"Going to your happy place" is something we often joke about, but there is some truth in the humor. Coussons-Read advises planning ahead and creating an internal picture of a place that relaxes you, so you can bring it to mind when you need it. Bedrooms and beaches top the list, but your happy site is a personal destination.

"Spend a little time creating what that picture looks like. When you feel stressed out, stop, put the picture in your head, take a few deep breaths," she says.

Pray

Prayer, in whatever form or from whatever tradition, can be a beneficial relaxation exercise. "It can have the component of relaxation but also the component of feeling part of something else, and feeling like you're not by yourself," she says.

Exercise

Being physically active on a regular basis is helpful for overall stress management, but if time allows, you can use physical exercise for immediate relaxation as well.

Taking a brief walk around your office building, doing some yoga stretches, or closing the door and dancing to a favorite tune can help alleviate stress. But "you don't want exercise to become just one more thing you have to do," says Coussons-Read, so pick something you enjoy.

Mini-massage

"One of the most important things is to recognize where and how you carry stress in your body–some carry it in shoulders, head, neck, jaw, hands or even their stomach," says Coussons-Read. Try scheduling an appointment with a massage therapist who can teach you how to take care of your trouble spots while at work or home.

Apply Heat

If you have the option of a warm bath or shower, or only have some warming gloves, socks, or heat packs, use the heat to help relax tight muscles.

Aromatherapy

Although research on aromatherapy is mixed, many people find certain scents, such as lavender to be relaxing. If you respond well to the smell, have a sample on hand (in a desk drawer or your purse) for a relaxing sniff as needed before or after your breathing exercises.

As hard as everyone works these days, we all deserve a time out now and then to calm our nerves and decompress. Relaxation exercises can help us stay productive and happy.

Burn Out

and

Stress Out

I'm not sure whether there is any comfort in the fact that the struggles that clergy are experiencing are not restricted to clergy in this country. I came upon an article on the same subject but from research done in Australia. In that article, the author made an interesting comparison between what it means to be stressed-out and burned-out.

DIFFERENCES BETWEEN

BURNOUT AND STRESS

Dr. Arch Hart

In the chart below, note the difference between the symptoms of burnout and stress. In each comparison, give yourself a rating. Mark S 1-10 and B 1-10 in each category. As you evaluate yourself, you may have a little of both in each area.

When you have finished, you can total your score for both burnout and stress.

BURNOUT	Two	STRESS
Give yourself a score from 1 to 10 in each box.	scores Burnout & Stress	Give yourself a score from 1 to 10 in each box.
Burnout is a defense characterized by disengagement.		Stress is characterized by over engagement.
In Burnout the emotions become blunted.		In Stress the emotions become over-reactive.
In Burnout the emotional damage is primary.		In Stress the physical damage is primary.
The exhaustion of Burnout affects motivation and drive.		The exhaustion of Stress affects physical energy.
Burnout produces demoralization.		Stress produces disintegration.
Burnout can best be understood as a loss		Stress can best be understood as a

of ideals and hope.		loss of fuel and energy.
The depression of Burnout is caused by grief engendered by the loss of ideals and hope.	81	The depression of Stress is produced by the body's need to protect itself and conserve energy
Burnout produces a sense of helplessness and hopelessness.		Stress produces a sense of urgency and hyperactivity.
Burnout produces paranoia, depersonalization and detachment.		Stress produces panic, phobic, and anxiety-type disorders.
Burnout may never kill you, but your long life may not seem worth living.		Stress may kill you prematurely, and you won't have enough time to finish what you started.

As you read this comparison, it becomes clear that burnout is more closely linked to spiritual issues while stress results from trying to do too much in too little time and not taking the necessary breaks. It is an excellent distinction to keep in mind.

When we experience stress, we need to deliberately take some recreative breaks. We can rest up and then continue. When we experience being burned out, we have lost the sense of meaning in our work. We need to reconnect with the source of our call.

Give yourself a rating in each area. How do you rate? When you total it up, you have a sense of how you need to focus.

Exercises to Relieve Stress

While I was at the compassion fatigue conference put on by PPCN, I picked up a little brochure put out by The

Fraser Center, www.frasercenter.com. In it was six anti-stress stretches that I pass on to you.

1 FINGER FAN: Extend your arms straight in front of you with palms up. Spread your fingers as far apart as possible. Hold for 5 seconds.

2.UPPER BACK STRETCH: Sit up straight with your fingers interlaced behind your head. Keeping your shoulders down, lift your chest and bring your elbows back as far as you can. Hold for 10 seconds.

3.EAR TO SHOULDER: Lower your right ear to your right shoulder. Hold for 10 seconds. Repeat on the other side.

4.OVERHEAD REACH: Raise your arms overhead and interlace your fingers with palms facing up. Keeping your shoulders down, stretch upwards. Hold for 20 seconds.

5.KNEE PULL: While seated bring one knee up toward your chest as high as possible. Hold with both hands for 10 seconds. Repeat for the other knee.

6.WAIST BEND: Reach arms overhead with fingers laced together. Facing forward with shoulders down, bend to one side from waist. Hold for 20 seconds. Repeat on the other side.

Does not sound too complicated, does it? I just went through these exercises, and it was easy. Now the trick is to remember to do them once an hour when you are working at a computer, after a counseling session, following a tough meeting, etc.

It does not make the challenges of life more comfortable, but it does help you prevent stress from robbing you of vital energy.

NOT GOOD

TO BE

ALONE

WHO DO I KNOW?

In his study of centenarians across the world, Dan Buettner discovered that a common factor was that these people had found their tribe. Each of them had become a part of a small group of friends who cared about them and held them accountable for being part of the living.

Genesis View of Humanity

When the Genesis story speaks of the creation of humanity, it suggests that creation included God´s recognition that it is not good for the human to be alone. From the beginning, the health of humans involved relationships. As the story unfolds in the rest of the journey of faith, it is clear that God is talking about more than just the relationship between men and women. All of faith is built on relationships. For Christians, that is summarized in the Great Commandment.

The suggestion in the story is that the relationships that give us health are more than just physical proximity. Pastors are surrounded by people. Many of those associations involve both physical and emotional interaction. However, as most pastors are fully aware, the profession of ministry can be a lonely profession. You respond to and interact with others, often on an emotional and even intense level, but the assumption is that the pastor is responding to the other person or group's emotions. Pastors always feel on stage and rarely are free to let their guard down.

In a survey of presbytery executives, almost all of them mentioned some version of loneliness and isolation as a chief issue for clergy. To paraphrase Genesis, "it is not good for clergy to be alone." If you apply the experience of centenarians to clergy, it does not contribute to their longevity as well. The challenge is that it is not easy for clergy to break through their isolation.

BEING INTENTIONAL AND PLAYFUL

Pastors have to be intentional but also playful about their need for companionship.

The **first step** is to recognize that taking time for healthy companionship can be a witness to others about the importance of friendship for everyone who seeks a healthy life. While one can exploit a relationship in a selfish, self-centered way, authentic relationships are part of a healthy ministry. Showing others how to balance productive efforts with re-creative relationships is vital to a healthy life.

The **second step** is to build a theological and preachable understanding of this balance. Your sermons can help your congregation to understand both yours and their need to nurture good relationships. For pastors, some of their friends need to be from outside the congregation. In publicly interpreting your intentionality to develop good relationships outside of professional responsibility, you are inviting the parishioners to hold you accountable as well as to see it as necessary for themselves. This is part of your ministry.

The **third step** is to seek playful ways to be with others. What are the types of experience that would be enjoyable, involve two or more people, and nurture the fruit of the Spirit within you? (Galatians 5:22-23) This can be done while playing golf, hiking, knitting, dancing, or going to a play.

Buettner found that people who live longest surround themselves with people who support healthy behaviors. Clergy need to develop a cadre of friends that help them have a healthy perspective on life and ministry. Ministry can be a complex quagmire that sucks you under. It is important to have some friends who both understand the challenges and the higher purpose to which you are called. With whom can you play and BE YOURSELF?

A DIFFERENT NEIGHBOR TO LOVE

IMPROVING THE NEIGHBORHOOD

Clergy have in their power the ability to have fun while improving the neighborhood. (If you are not a pastor, pass this along as a fun invitation.) Look around your community and note and identify four or five churches who have at least one full-time pastor. Be bold and select churches of different denominations or no denomination, liberal and conservative. Find out the name and contact information for the pastor.

AN INVITATION

Prepare to write each a letter that will be followed up with a phone call. (These days a letter is far more effective than an email.) Explain that since you are pastoring in the same neighborhood, you would like to become better acquainted. Towards that end, you would like to call them in the next several days and invite them, along with a few other neighbor pastors to choose an afternoon when you could all go to a movie and share a light meal afterward to both discuss the movie and become familiar with each other's ministry.

NO HIDDEN AGENDA

Assure them that you have no hidden agenda or any expectation of any action beyond a shared awareness that as clergy we share a stressful calling and occasionally can offer personal support in a too often fractured world. Also, tell them that you recognize that we come from diverse theological perspectives, but you affirm with Paul "there are varieties of gifts, but the same Spirit." (1 Cor 12:4)

SUGGEST A MOVIE

Pick out a movie that you think might be appealing, identify the times for a late afternoon matinee, and a nearby restaurant. I suggest that a Monday or Tuesday or Friday afternoon might work best. Tell them you will call them in the next couple of days to hear their response. When you do call, be prepared for some hesitation. If they say that they have a conflict, ask whether they would be open to a future time or even a different venue.

LOVE YOUR NEIGHBOR

What you are doing is beginning to build community among pastors in your neighborhood. Not everyone will be willing to join you, but if you can get between three and five, you have a good start. Consider it an adventure into the unknown that will likely have some pleasant and unexpected results. It is a specific act of "loving your neighbor."

GO AHEAD,

TAKE A CHANCE,

IT COULD BE FUN.

HEALTHY CLERGY IS A LAUGHING MATTER

"MAKE LAUGHTER A HABIT"

By Katherine Zeratsky, R.D., L.D. and Jennifer K. Nelson, R.D., L.D.

Laughter is about being present. When you laugh, you enjoy the here and now. There are therapeutic benefits to laughter and, for this reason, it is one of the 12 Habits of Highly Healthy People. Research shows laughter offers us health benefits in four health dimensions: physical, intellectual, emotional, and spiritual.

Physical Health

- Laughter is like "internal jogging." It temporarily increases your heart rate and blood pressure, followed by muscle relaxation and a decrease in blood pressure.

- It may boost the immune system and promote healing.

- It burns calories–60 to 120 calories an hour over your resting metabolism.

Intellectual Health

- Laughter can create a positive effect which influences attention, institution, creativity, and imagination.

- It can enhance employee morale, resilience, and belief in one's abilities in the workplace.

Emotional Health

- Laughter is a tremendous constructive coping skill.

- It can reduce stress by providing a positive way to look at a problem.

- It solidifies friendships and makes people feel included.

Spiritual Health

- Laughter is a universal language and can be an interfaith experience. It fosters connection and compassion.

OTHER OPPORTUNITIES:

1. Try laughter yoga—a fun combination of stretching, breathing, and laughing exercises that can help you feel awakened, confident, creative, productive, and ready to tackle anything http://www.laughinglaura.com.

2. Build an inventory of funny jokes, cartoons, and stories.

3. Have a joke jar at home or in your office.

It's important to distinguish between laughter that heals and laughter that hurts. Consider how you can bring more gratitude, acceptance, and laughter into your life and lives of those you touch.

BE SERIOUS ENOUGH

TO LAUGH

While Dan Buttner, in his study of centenarians, does not mention humor as a significant factor in their longevity, I think it is a critical factor in healthy ministry. If you cannot laugh at yourself and some of the crazy situations you find in the ministry, you are putting yourself under far more stress than is healthy. Ministry is a serious business, but a good laugh can make space for God to do even better work through you and your church.

Judy Carter, one of my favorite comedians, who I was able to interview in my book *God Laughs–Why Don't You?*, suggests that a significant stress reduction strategy is to learn how to turn your problems into punch lines bit.ly/Godlaughs.

PROBLEMS INTO PUNCHLINES

When someone comes up with that tired old doggerel, "It must be nice to work only one hour a week," wouldn't it be nice to respond with something like, "I only wish I could take the other sixty-nine hours off my taxes as a charitable donation."

Or when someone thinks he's being wise and intones, "What I want to know is when you clergy are going to understand that the church needs to be run like a business. You need to get your head out of the clouds." Would you like to respond, "Having read about the mess that a lot of corporations have created, I wonder if your recommendation would include a golden parachute if I mess up."

A DIARY OF HUMOR

For lots of reasons, you may not feel free to come back with such responses directly. Though lots of times, about an hour later, you think of what you would have liked to have said.

First, get yourself a notebook and copy down the whiny or mean-spirited comments you hear. Make a list of the unfair criticism that you at times absorb with a smile. Then, when you are alone, try to make the best ripposte you can think of. Believe me; you will get better the more you do it. I guarantee you that there will be occasions that it will lift your spirits to go back and read some of them.

Second, find one or two colleagues in the ministry. Covenant with them to once a month send your best retorts to each other. Shared humor is healing.

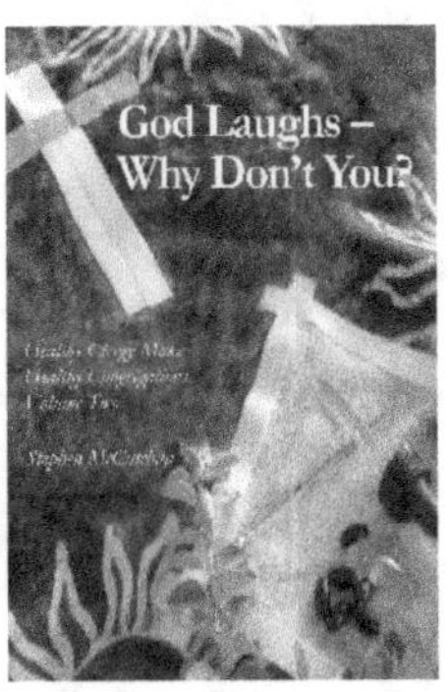

<u>bit.ly/Godlaughs</u>

My book attempts to share several strategies about how to integrate humor into ministry. I take ministry seriously, which is why I needed to learn to laugh.

USE

FICTION

FOR HEALTH

A STORY OF YOUR FUTURE

Have you ever wondered where you will be five or ten years from now? Would you like a safe way to look into the future? I'm sure that you have occasionally had a fantasy about some future possibility—or maybe even a nightmare. What if you can look into several futures so that you can choose from among them.

You are invited to try fiction to explore possible futures. You do not have to be a great writer to engage in putting possibilities into a story form. Choose either a pen and paper or more likely a computer and paint a picture of one or more possible futures.

DON'T TAKE YOUR TIME

The two biggest excuses for not doing this are:

1. I don't know how to write fiction.

2. I don't have time to do this.

Do not allow either of these excuses to prevent you from having an enjoyable adventure. You have told stories before–not all of them accurate–and this time you do not have to feel guilty. Since you are the primary audience of your account, you do not need to worry about writing skills.

Concerning the issue of time, I would suggest both short and long possibilities. Once you get started, you may find time to extend your effort, but even short stories have an impact. Look how powerful some of the parables are.

So, find an hour and be prepared for some enlightening fun.

"WHAT IF"

IS ALL YOU NEED

The scene for your story is a meeting ten years in the future with two close friends who are meeting you for a leisurely dinner and good conversation. You can try it either way, but it might be interesting to have one male and one female friend for this conversation. If you do, try to be conscious of how the perspective is affected by being either a male or a female.

It is ten years in the future, and you are looking back on the significant events over the last ten years and your current physical condition. I think you will find it easiest if you write this as a dialogue. Allow your companions to raise questions and probe your story.

Begin by describing your physical health—good or bad—maybe even in crisis mode. In conversation with your friends, describe what behavior, decisions, events beyond your control, etc. have resulted in both your physical and emotional health.

Describe three decisions that you think now had a significant effect on your current health condition. Do not overthink this. Begin writing and try not to stop for at least a half-hour. I think you will be surprised at what unfolds.

In short, you are telling stories about possible futures that might occur for you. By writing them down, they become a more concrete way of exploring potential consequences of decisions you make in your life.

By beginning your dialogue by describing to your fictional friends your physical and emotional health and the decisions about lifestyle, behavior, and relationships that have led you to this condition in your life, you are exploring consequences. By writing them down in a dialogue with fictional friends, it makes the decisions more real.

You may find it fun to choose several scenarios where you have arrived at different conditions.

Now begin to explain to your fictional friends how these decisions in the last ten years have had a significant impact on how your life evolved. Help them understand why you made these decisions and how these decisions affected you. You can explore what you now see as bad or even foolish choices, or you can choose to describe wise or intelligent decisions. In either case, try to be realistic regarding the people who surround you and how they would react. Don't explain the end results but tell how different people reacted and perhaps why they responded that way.

GOOD FRIENDS LOVE STORIES

Once you have tried this a couple of times, you might want to invite a couple of good friends to engage in a similar process and then share and talk about your stories. Listening to their stories might stimulate some

alternative possibilities for you as well.

CONGREGATIONS

SUPPORT

THEIR CLERGY

Support Your Clergy

There is a difference between pampering your clergy and demonstrating care and support for their ministry. If a congregation is going to expect someone to perform excellent work in a demanding profession, knowing how to offer support and appreciation for their work can enhance their performance. If you reflect on the time and emotional cost of searching for and adjusting to a new clergy, it makes sense to keep your clergy and staff physically and emotionally healthy.

In this book, we focus on strategies to support the physical health of the clergy and staff. Three major areas that attend to a person's physical health are those of exercise, diet, and sleep. A fourth area to address in both the category of physical health and emotional health is that of how a person responds to stress.

A task force of the leadership can reflect, first by themselves and then with the clergy, on how the practice of ministry can affect a clergy's physical health. This is not because there is something the congregation is doing wrong, but it is being aware of the nature of ministry in our time.

Some behavior that might contribute to poor health:

1. Lack of a dedicated time to do physical exercise.

2. Not belonging to a Y or sports club where they have the exercise equipment.

3. Not participating in a sport or communal activity involving physical activity.

4. Not getting regular physical exams that monitor health.

5. Skipping or rushing meals because of professional demands.

6. Not having a good awareness of healthy foods.

7. Not monitoring one's weight.

8. Poor sleep habits.

9. Not allowing enough time for sleep.

10. Being aware of ways to interrupt stress when it has built up.

11. Recognizing and allowing for situations that trigger negative emotional responses.

12. Add areas from your group discussion.

Share your list with the clergy and see if there are other areas that emerge from the discussion.

Following that discussion, the group can discuss how they might help the clergy address some of these areas.

Begin with one or two items on the list and then agree to meet again in a few months to attend to other areas. The process will raise awareness of the concern and build support for the health of the clergy and for others as well.

A helpful approach might be to share the concern with the congregation and invite others to join in a mutual focus on physical health.

Congregational Support of the Health of Staff

Consider some specific strategies that the leadership of a congregation might take:

First, the leadership can become familiar with the wellness program offered by the Board of Pensions of the Presbyterian Church (U.S.A.) at www.pensions.org. Here is an example of the value of the connectional church.

Second, express support for the pastor and others on the staff to maintain their physical health. Be sure they are aware of the resources of the Board of Pensions.

Third, a congregation can support their staff in taking the time to make physical exercise a part of their routine. One church had a member that offered use of his weight machines for the pastor's use. Several congregations have tried to help provide membership at a Y or sports club. In some cases, the health insurance will even help with the cost of such a membership.

Fourth, since people are often reluctant to intrude on a person's personal physical life, an entry point might be to invite the pastor and educator to lead the whole congregation in reflecting on the spiritual dimensions of physical health. According to Paul (1 Corinthians 19), this is a spiritual issue for the entire Body of Christ.

HAVING THE HEALTH CARE CONVERSATION

Recognizing that the elders or deacons of a congregation are also part of the spiritual leadership of the church, begin by having the health conversation with the whole board. On the agenda set aside some time to reflect on the health challenges facing the leadership of the congregation. Ask all the individuals to talk about the health challenges facing many members of their congregation. Make a list as they are identified. For example, people are overweight, some don't exercise enough, they don't get enough sleep, they drink too much, and others. The conversation raises the consciousness about the subject before it gets personal.

Next, engage in a brief reflection on the faith issues that speak to our care of our physical bodies. Explore the connection between our religious journey and our health journey. What is it in our faith that speaks to our care of our bodies. Develop a brief confession on the connection between physical health and faithfulness.

Then pass out some blank 4 x 6 cards. Tell all the members that you are going to have a time of silent prayer in which each is asked to reflect on and identify an action that they think if they did it regularly would contribute to their health. At the end of the prayer time, they are to write down on both halves of the card the action they identified but without placing their names on the cards. They then tear the card in half, keeping one half and turning in the other.

The cards are compiled into a list to share at the next meeting. At that next session, each member is asked to rate how they have done this past month in taking the action that would contribute to their health using a scale of 1–10 with 10 representing complete success.

Each month, for a year, at their regular meeting, the same procedure should be followed, and a graph of success recorded for each area. After each time of sharing, there is a time of prayer in which the person rededicates him or herself to practicing their designated action for the year. The church staff, as well as the leadership, are included in this communal effort to address the physical health of our journey of faith.

INCLUDE THE CONGREGATION

IN THE DISCUSSION

Many times problems in the ministry can be converted to possibilities if they are reframed. We can make the noblest of excuses for our failure to take care of our health because we are too busy taking care of others. However, the problem of declining physical health is not restricted to pastors but is rampant in our society. It would not be difficult to translate some of our society's problem with declining health as an issue of poor stewardship of the bodies that God has provided us. A few well-developed sermons on this aspect of stewardship could result in raising a congregational awareness as to the connection between our faith and caring for our bodies.

The next step would be to engage the congregation in exercising their imagination concerning ways that physical activities can be incorporated into congregational events.

One day could be devoted to cleaning the church building in a way that involved conscious exercise movements. Perhaps some vigorous rhythmic music could encourage some extra movement.

A neighborhood walk can be planned in which each person has a litter bag and the contest would be to see who could gather the most litter and leave the neighborhood in better condition.

A group can be tasked with designing healthier meals for the next congregational supper and maybe include some mild stretching exercises as part of the evening.

If there is a large fellowship hall, a sports night with a variety of fun activities for the non-sports-experts can be planned.

The whole congregation can be invited to see who could come up with the most creative ways for the community to have some exercise during their congregational events.

Then, throughout the year, people's progress in finding new ways to exercise can be publicly celebrated.

THE LARGER

CHURCH

SUPPORTS

THEIR CLERGY

ENCOURAGE MEMBERS OF JUDICATORY TO:

1. Call a clergy colleague, invite him or her to lunch, ask them to tell you about his or her ministry and then listen.

2. Plan to attend conferences that focus on clergy health. The Board of Pensions may be able to identify some possibilities.

3. Sign up for the PPCN newsletter (free on request) and continue to get regular practical suggestions on clergy health. The newsletter is issued about five times a year with suggestions for clergy, churches, and judicatories. The health plan of most denominations has similar information.

4. Subscribe and share ideas from my blog, www.smccutchan.com, for more ideas about how the church and clergy can contribute to keeping clergy healthy. Send me questions and comments, and I will try to respond.

5. Identify three clergy of different churches and pray for them and their ministry for 30 days in a row. (If you miss a day, add two days at the end.)

6. It is a discipline from which both you and the clergy will benefit.

Bonus:

7. Laughter is good for the soul. Complete the following sentence three times. Share it with a colleague:

"Clergy must be crazy if they . . ."

1.

2.

3.

Go ahead, have a little fun, enjoy some laughter, and know that God gave us a sense of humor to be an antidote to the stresses of life.

INTRODUCING THE TOPIC TO CHURCHES IN THE JUDICATORY

FIVE REASONS YOU CARE ABOUT HEALTHY CLERGY & WHAT TO DO ABOUT IT

You care about clergy because:

1. You believe that God calls clergy to ministry

    A divine source sparked their choice of ministry.

2. You understand the demanding nature of the ministry.

> Both the physical and emotional demands of ministry take their cumulative toll.

3. You care about your colleagues in ministry.

> They are neighbors that need signs of compassion from time to time.

4. You know that Healthy Clergy Make Healthy Congregations.

> When clergy are healthy physically, emotionally, and spiritually, they are more likely to shape a healthy congregation.

5. You see how healthy congregations contribute to a better world.

> Have them suggest one action a church board could take in support of the church staff.

Pass out the sheet of FIVE REASONS and have both the lay members and the clergy each choose from the list their top two choices. After the selection is made, have them discuss their choices in small groups that include both lay and clergy.

Have the lay members and the clergy identify at least one action a church board can take in support of the church staff.

INTRODUCING

CLERGY HEALTH

This is an exercise that a judicatory might use to introduce the subject of clergy health to clergy and lay members. Copy the time chart and distribute it to all who are present at the meeting.

HOW WELL DO YOU KNOW YOUR

MINISTER(S), EDUCATOR(S)

Below is a list of tasks that the minister or educator performs regularly. Lay members guess the number of hours they think might be required in the average week of ministry. Guessing is allowed and even encouraged. Ministers/educators likewise estimate the number of hours spent.

MINISTRY TIME CHART

TELEPHONE, E-MAIL, CORRESPONDENCE _______

ADMINISTRATION _______

SUPERVISION OF STAFF &/OR VOLUNTEERS _______

COMMITTEE MEETINGS DURING THE DAY _______

COMMITTEE MEETINGS HELD AT NIGHT _______

WORSHIP PLANNING AND CONDUCTING _______

SERMON PREPARATION AND PREACHING _______

PRIVATE PRAYER AND SPIRITUAL PRACTICE _______

CHURCH SCHOOL PLANNING _______

TEACHER / OFFICER TRAINING _______

HOSPITAL OR CRISIS VISITING _______

HOME VISITING _______

TEACHING _______

COUNSELING _______

SPECIAL EVENT PLANNING & PARTICIPATION _______
(weddings, funerals, seasonal events,)

YOUTH MINISTRY _______

CHILDREN'S MINISTRY _______

SERVICE & MISSION WORK _______

COMMUNITY WORK WITH OTHER CHURCHES _______

EVANGELISM AND WITNESS _______

DENOMINATIONAL WORK _______

*****

TOTAL HOURS =====

Once everyone has had a chance to fill out their sheet, have small groups discuss the results with mixtures of clergy and lay people.

EMOTIONAL ROLLER COASTER

We recognize that clergy are engaged in highly emotional situations. Not only negative situations but highly satisfactory experiences can take their toll on a pastor's energy levels. Compassion fatigue can easily result from continually seeking to respond to the needs of others. The better and more compassionate a pastor is, the more s/he is subject to these conditions. Add to that the need to also engage in an almost continuous series of routine activities that are demanding of time and energy but not very stimulating and you have some sense of the emotional roller-coaster nature of ministry.

Using the time chart and your imagination, try to picture the variety of activities that your pastor might engage in over a three-month period. On a scale of 1–10, using both positive and negative numbers to represent both positive and negative emotions, try to picture the emotional ride of being a pastor. For example, I visit a terminal patient and that is a negative 5. I celebrate with a couple the birth of their new child and that is a positive 6. Not every week has a baptism, a tragic accident, a marital counseling session, a negative or positive response to a sermon, teaching the confirmation class, trying to manage a budget deficit, and so on. Try to build in some typical possibilities that might occur over three months' time. Notice the emotional demands. Then think about this not being for just a few months or even a couple of years but continually moving through this emotional roller-coaster.

After the group has discussed their findings, ask for a discussion about the church's interest in exploring possible strategies to combat the physical stress of ministry. This can be the basis to explore with its members a strategy to address the health issues of ministry through a variety of future events.

REGIONAL STRATEGIES

Since we are facing some shocking statistics on the decline of clergy health, it is vital that judicatories, in our case presbyteries, look at what they can do to encourage clergy to take care of themselves physically. What follows are some scattered ideas to motivate judicatories to begin to think creatively in this area.

1. Occasionally have some simple health screening available at gatherings. Even as basic as inviting a parish nurse to offer blood pressure tests, body mass index, carotid artery scans.

2. Weight loss contests can be set up–somewhat based on the Biggest Loser TV program.

3. Congregations can compete with each other to see who could come up with the best health maintenance program. The Lutherans (ECLA) have encouraged a denomination-wide plan to lift up great congregational programs for health.

4. A health checkup list can be developed and sent to the sessions of the congregations listing some basic practices–exercise, sufficient sleep, healthy eating practices, that the pastor and session can discuss as a communal effort to nurture the health of the leadership.

5. Visit ;your medical plan website to learn about wellness resources and make these resources available at judicatory meetings.

6. Invite a representative from the Board of Pensions or your medical plan to offer a seminar on the various wellness programs during a judicatory leadership event or mission fair.

7. Some of the programs offered by the Board of Pensions to encourage good health can be identified for the churches so that they can take advantage of them.

8. There are programs on:

1. Weight loss,

2. Smoking cessation,

3. Chronic illness management, etc.

If such programs were spread out over several meetings, it would also create a cultural awareness of the importance of physical health that could benefit the whole judicatory. This might lead to other discussions and other programs that will assist in maintaining a healthy church. To paraphrase Paul, "If one pastor suffers, all suffer together." (1 Corinthians 12:26)

HEALTH FAIR

AN ECUMENICAL WITNESS TO THE COMMUNITY

Consider an action several churches in the same neighborhood could take to address the health issue. It will be a positive witness to the broader community if executives from the various denominations in an area coordinated to offer a health fair for clergy and professional staff. Make sure to include some nondenominational community churches as well.

An excellent guide for planning a health fair can be found at

_http://www.rockteach.org/sites/default/files/Guide_fo_

_r_

_Planning_a_Health_Fair.pdf_

A local branch of a large health insurance industry like Blue Cross might help sponsor such an event. By doing it ecumenically, or even interfaith, you can have sufficient numbers not to have anyone drive too far. Plus, you probably can get some good media coverage for a positive, cooperative event among the churches.

The first step would be to approach a local hospital and talk with them about providing health personnel for such an event. If you are near an educational, medical center, they probably have a division that will be glad to work with you on designing such an event.

At the event, you can offer to **check**:

1. Blood pressure.

2. Glucose level.

3. Cholesterol level.

4. Weight.

Demonstrate:

1. Mouth-to-mouth resuscitation

2. Use of a defibrillator

3. Seminars on healthy cooking

4. Home exercise programs,

5. Stress reduction programs

An additional advantage for the pastor is that s/he would be better informed about what to do if a member of the congregation showed such symptoms.

Because your focus is on pastors and professional church staff, it would be good to have some elements built into the design that address the unique aspects of working in a church and the resultant pressures of such a profession.

If the health fair is successful, several neighboring congregations might be encouraged to join together to offer a similar festival for their membership.

BEYOND PUTTING OUT FIRES

I have invited Alan Baroody to share some suggestions that the Committee on Ministry or Pastoral Care Committee might implement as a proactive action on behalf of the clergy in your region: Some of these are repetitive of suggestions in other sections of this book.

- Make use of and promote Board of Pension and denominational resources for clergy wellness.

- Make available clergy support groups and clergy spouse support groups.

- Contract with local resources to provide confidential counseling.

- Encourage "Facebook" or other online support/interest groups.

- Write boundary expectations into Calls and Covenants for clergy whereby the congregation agrees that a pastor's spending time with spouse and family is expected, days off are protected, and participation in the activities and leadership within the local community are encouraged.

- Either in the church's call or the regional budget, have funds available for clergy recreational activities or hobbies.

- Form a pastoral care team and/or have a designated pastor-to-pastors and chaplain for clergy spouses.

- Be creative in sponsoring clergy retreats and outings (cruises, fishing contests, golf matches, tickets to concerts and civic events, tours or trips).

- Arrange for corporate contract membership fees for YMCAs and health clubs within the bounds of the judicatory.

- Sponsor health fairs and wellness contests for clergy and their families.

- Form a mentor-colleague program with means for accountability to make sure contacts are being made.

(Don't forget retired pastors and ministers serving in setting other than the local congregation.)

- Develop a "First Call" program for new clergy retention and wellness.

- Sponsor annual clergy and clergy-spouse retreats.

- Consider sponsoring quarterly district luncheons.

- Acknowledge clergy anniversaries, birthdays, ordination dates, etc.

- Sponsor continuing education workshops and courses for clergy that have nothing to do with congregational ministry (beginners golf or tennis lessons, foreign language series, "how to" water ski, fish, snow ski, bowl, sail, bird-watch. Use your imagination!)

- Make sure spiritual resources are available and their use encouraged by clergy and their spouses.

- Sponsor movie/theater/concert groups.

The healthier you keep your clergy, the less committee time you will spend on putting out fires.

Alan Baroody na4nb@yahoo.com

Helping Pastors who are Depressed

Studies indicate a rise in depression among the clergy. The first things for a judicatory or congregation to recognize are the signs of depression. Depression is a medical condition, but inappropriate attitudes and responses can exacerbate it. A pastor who is experiencing this condition is under enormous pressure to both deny it personally and to hide it from others.

The following symptoms, when they occur nearly every day for at least two weeks, are solid indicators that a person needs help:

- Depressed mood most of the day; feeling sad or empty, tearful.
- Significant loss of interest or pleasure in activities that used to be enjoyable.

- Significant weight loss (when not dieting) or weight gain; decrease or increase in appetite.

- Difficulty sleeping or sleeping too much.

- Agitation; or slowing down of thoughts and reduction of physical movements.

- Fatigue or loss of energy.

- Feelings of worthlessness or inappropriate guilt.

- Poor concentration or having difficulty making decisions.

- Thinking about death or suicide.

It is very scary to have any of these symptoms. It is enormously helpful for clergy to know that there is a safe place where they can explore what they are experiencing.

Depression is a severe physical and mental reality, and we need to mature in our ability to be supportive of each other.

Unhelpful Versus Helpful Responses to a

Depressed Colleague

I'm sure it must be true for others as well, but clergy can experience a large measure of guilt when they are depressed. That guilt compounds their sense of isolation and helplessness. Consider some of the central messages of the Christian faith that counter unhelpful responses that they can both hear and internalize.

In the place of, "It always helps me to remember that there are people far worse off than I am.", they need to hear something like, "You are an important part of the Body of Christ, and we are here for you."

Instead of "Stop feeling sorry for yourself, no one said life was fair," they need to hear, "I don't want you to feel alone as you struggle with this. Let's explore together how God might work through this with you."

Instead of, "If you just had enough faith, this wouldn't be a problem for you," or "Why do you think God is punishing you at this time," they need to hear, "Depression is real." You are not crazy, and it's not your fault."

Instead of "I once had a friend who was depressed, and he was helped by (whatever home remedy you've heard about)," they need to hear, "You need to get a competent medical diagnosis, and if you want, I will go with you to the appointment."

Instead of, "Buck up, you'll feel better in a few days" or "Just try to think positive," they need to hear, "I can't possibly understand what you are feeling, but I do believe God works best with wounded healers. As painful as this is, we can all grow from this if you will let us accompany you on this journey."

WE

CAN

HAVE A PLAN

PLAN NOW TO BE HEALTHY

Make clergy aware of health resources. These resources are from the Presbyterian Board of Pensions.

https://www.pensions.org

Other denominations have similar resources.

Preventative Health Care

Studies show that good preventive care reduces health care costs, improves medical outcomes, and even saves lives. That's why there's no office co-pay for annual wellness visits for benefits plan members if they are network primary care physicians and gynecologists. Be sure to give your doctor an up-to-date preventive schedule that shows the screenings, tests, and immunizations that are covered for your age group. This plan is available on the Website at *www.pensions.org* Call the Board of Pensions to request the preventive schedule (800-773-7752)

Manage Your Health Condition

Get help from ActiveHealth Management of the Board of Pensions for many chronic diseases or conditions. Through the health management program, Informed Care Management, you'll be assigned a nurse who will work with you over the phone as your health coach. Your nurse coach can help you make smart choices about treating and controlling your health issues. By working with a nurse, you may be able to delay the onset of complications—or even avoid them altogether.

Keep in mind that you don't have to be sick to call the 24-Hour Nurse Line, a hotline provided through ActiveHealth Management. You can speak with an experienced, registered nurse at any time about your health concerns. For for more information, contact ActiveHealth call 866-794-3127.

YOUR NURSE WILL:

- Answer your questions

- Send you specific information about your health concerns

- Review warning signs to watch for

- Advise you on topics to discuss with your doctor

When you work with a nurse through the Informed Care Management Program, he or she typically will schedule calls with you about four times a year. These calls are not a substitute for a visit to the doctor. They are intended to help you work more effectively with your doctor and avoid future complications.

CONDITIONS INCLUDED AS PART OF THIS PROGRAM ARE:

1. Heart and blood vessel conditions

2. Diabetes

3. Lung conditions

4. Stomach and intestine conditions

5. Kidney conditions

6. Cancer

7. Bone and joint conditions

8. Neurologic conditions

9. Cystic fibrosis

10. HIV

11. Sickle cell anemia

PROGRAMS ALSO ARE AVAILABLE FOR CHILDREN AND TEENS WITH THE FOLLOWING CONDITIONS:

- Asthma

- Diabetes

- Cystic fibrosis

- High blood pressure

- Sickle cell anemia

- Weight management/obesity

Your medical benefits include a confidential Case Management Program, provided by ActiveHealth. This program helps you when you have frequent or prolonged hospital admissions, require ongoing healthcare services in your home, or need continuing care in outpatient settings. Case Management helps members get the best available treatment when underlying health conditions may be complicated or challenging to address.

The program can assist you by:

- Helping you understand the resources available to you.

- Coordinating and helping arrange medical services for you.

- Providing education and support for you and your family.

A nurse will work with you and your physician to facilitate approval for medically necessary services under the provisions of the Medical Plan. Your nurse will also help evaluate treatment needs and options under the direction of your attending physician. Contact ActiveHealth Management: 866-794-3127

THE GIFT

OF AN

INTERIM

PASTOR

A UNIQUE

OPPORTUNITY

A significant problem in raising a congregation's awareness concerning the health of clergy is "Who can raise the question?" Clergy are reluctant to talk about it because it seems to be self-serving. It's even difficult for sessions to raise it for discussion because they don't want to suggest that the pastor is somehow weak and needs pampering. Plus, though they are in the leadership of the church, they don't fully understand the particular pressures in a pastor's life.

Consider the unique position an interim can play in educating a congregation. First, s/he speaks from the perspective of a pastor. Second, s/he is focused on what can be done to help both the congregation and the future pastor to be healthy.

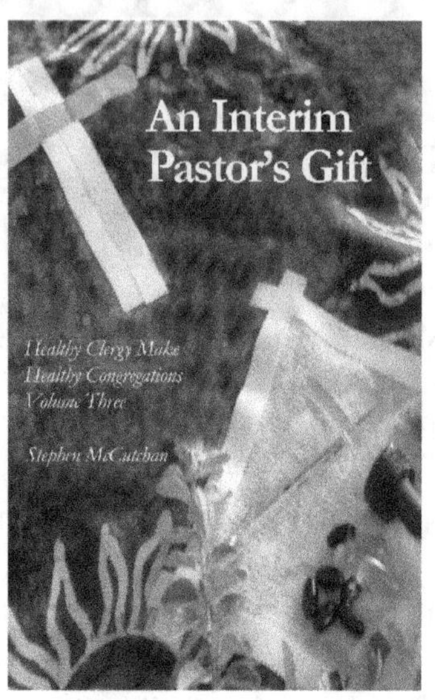

The judicatory can provide the interim with a booklet

bit.ly/InterimGift that will offer a strategy for the

education of the congregation.

BEFORE A CANDIDATE IS SELECTED

Even before a specific candidate is identified, the interim can guide the session in reflecting on the challenges of the ministry that affect the health of clergy. What are the factors that might contribute to the dramatic decline in physical health among clergy? The Duke Health Initiative found that 79% of Methodists clergy in North Carolina had problems with obesity. The study also showed that the depression rate among the clergy was significantly higher than the average population. The leadership can discuss the factors in ministry that can contribute to physical and emotional stress, family health, spiritual health, financial stress, etc.

SECONDARY STRESS

Both the pastor and the session need to recognize that we are not talking about weakness but strength in the ministry. The better a pastor is, the more s/he will be sensitive to and therefore absorb the pain of the congregation. Studies have shown that a person who genuinely listens to another person's pain absorbs some of that pain into themselves. The result is an increase in the stress in the person's life. A good pastor will be responsive to the wide-ranging pain of the congregation but rarely has a chance to recover from the trauma in one person's life before they confront the pain is several more people. In most cases, it is not even a pain that they can share and receive support. How do you say, "I'm feeling devastated by a marriage I see breaking up before my eyes?" Members will reach out to the affected family, but they rarely think about the pastor who has born that secret for a period of time.

By raising these questions for public discussion before a specific person is involved, the leadership can begin to strategize on how to be supportive of their new pastor.

HAVING A PRECLERGY CONVERSATION

An interim, who knows the various excuses that busy pastors give for not caring for themselves, can assist the session or governing body in thinking through this issue. When the interim offers advice before a specific pastor is identified, personalities are not involved, and the value the congregation places on clergy health is declared.

AN EXERCISE FOR THE SESSION

From the list below, identify at least one area where your congregation is already supporting clergy and staff and one where they could do a better job.

We encourage our pastor(s) and staff to:

1. Have a dedicated time to do physical exercise.

2. Belong to a Y or sports club where they have exercise equipment and trainers.

3. Participate in a sport or some other communal activity that engages in physical activity.

4. Get annual physical exams.

5. Avoid skipping or rushing meals because of professional demands

6. Not answer the phone during family dinners but use the voice mail.

7. Be aware of healthy foods and a proper diet.

8. Monitor one's weight.

9. Have good sleep habits.

10. Allow for enough time for sleep.

11. Be aware of ways to interrupt stress when it has increased to a high level.

12. Recognize and make allowances for situations that trigger negative emotional responses.

Once the leadership has identified several areas that seem appropriate for their congregation, they can consider how they want to communicate this concern as the search committee narrows in on a particular candidate.

A CONVERSATION WITH THE NEW PASTOR

Then, when a new pastor is identified, church committee is prepared to have discussions with the new pastor about ways that they can be supportive of his or her health— physical, emotional, family, financial, spiritual, and vocational. Imagine the positive impression a congregation can make by being proactive in asking the pastor to be a good steward of the pastor's health.

One strategy might be for the committee to say to the new pastor, "Over the next six months we want you to examine one of these areas each month and discuss with us how both the pastor and the congregation can address this issue." As a resource for the pastor, they can provide him or her with some of the volumes in this series for reflection.

BUILDING A THEOLOGICAL FRAMEWORK

An additional contribution that the interim can make is to spend the last several Sundays in the pulpit addressing various issues of the stewardship of health. The issues raised concern the health of the entire Christian community and particularly its leadership. By using several sermons to address the topic, the interim can provide the theological framework by which the whole church can be conscious of the importance of maintaining good health.

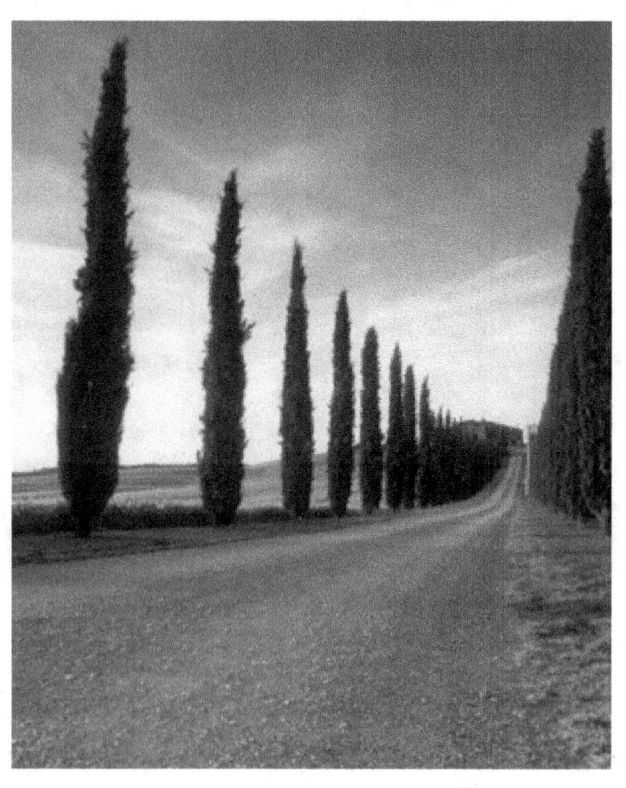

RETIREMENT

THIRD PHASE OF LIFE

Regardless of your age or how long you plan to continue before retirement, I encourage you to compose some fictional pictures of what you will do in retirement. Consider several possible scenes.

One scenario might be a retirement party and what people will say about your ministry.

Another might be what exciting new life might evolve for you in your retirement.

Most of our future is the result of our decisions much earlier, so therefore I encourage you to explore those possibilities now and be prepared to take actions that offer positive outcomes.

Disciplines for

Retirement

When pastors retire from active ministry, it is easy for us to let our adjustment to a new lifestyle also alter some of the disciplines that are good for us. This is true in all six areas of health in the series Healthy Clergy Make Healthy Congregations. This book gives attention to the disciplines that focus on physical health.

While there are many physical health problems that can occur with advancing age, there are several that seem to haunt all of us. As a **first step**, jot down a list of some of the physical challenges that might face you as you advance in age. Take advantage of your experience as a pastor and recall what many of your parishioners have experienced. Your list might include such things as diabetes, strokes, heart attacks, and forms of dementia. List at least ten to push you beyond the obvious.

In many ways, you can't prevent your body from confronting these problems, but there are things you can do that should help. If something comes along that you could not have prevented, then you deal with it. However, if it is something that you could have avoided, then you bear some responsibility for your condition.

As a **second step**, look at your list of ten and make one or two statements in each area of things you can do that may lessen the threat of that concern. For example, in your retirement, you need to pay attention to your diet.

Be an advocate of moderation and occasional exceptions in looking at your diet but don't ignore the obvious.

You need to keep track of the various indicators of problems such as high cholesterol, high blood pressure, etc. One thing you need to do is get regular check-ups with your primary care physician.

You need to be aware of what you eat, keep it balanced, and not overindulge. Since being overweight is a contributing factor for many problems, you need to monitor this continually. That doesn't mean you can't have some extras now and then, but overall you need to pay attention—even more so in your later years than in earlier times.

Then There Is Exercise.

You need to:

1. Find some sport or game that you can share with others that is both fun and helps the heartbeat.

2. Be intentional about a weight and stretching program.

3. Schedule walks more frequently.

These are just examples. There are other physical things that you can do. Use your imagination and identify as many as you can. You won't do all of them, but as your life changes, having the list will be an excellent resource.

HAVE A HEALTH CONVERSATION WITH A RETIRED COLLEAGUE

Find a colleague with whom you can explore the questions listed below. Not all will apply, but choose those that fit your situation.

QUESTIONS FOR CONSIDERATION:

1. Do you get a yearly physical checkup with a doctor?

2. Do you have a regular exercise program that includes both a strength component and a cardio component?

3. Do you participate in a sport that helps you stay in shape?

4. Evaluate your diet. Do you limit your intake of unhealthy foods?

5. Is your weight within some healthy margin?

6. Do you belong to a Y or sports club that encourages you to exercise?

7. Do you have a home exercise machine?

8. Do you participate in yoga, Tai Chi, Pilate, or some other stretch and relax program?

9. Do you have a partner(s) that help you stay accountable for your exercising?

10. Are you part of either a running or walking regimen?

11. Do you have a mini-exercise routine that you can use when you are traveling or limited in time?

12. Do you know how to practice meditation or relaxation breathing when you are under stress?

13. Are you aware of signs of stress in your body that alert you to the need to reduce your level of stress?

14. Are you familiar with some basic first aid if you should experience injury?

15. Do you get sufficient sleep to restore your body?

16. Are you aware of specific relaxation techniques when you have trouble sleeping?

17. Do you have a good breakfast every day?

Your physical health in retirement is significant. Before you conclude your conversation identify, some of the ways you might build a covenant with your colleague to improve your physical health. Accountability will help you take action.

FINAL WORD

Since my retirement in 2006, I've had the privilege of serving the church in a new way by focusing on developing resources that can assist clergy, congregations, and judicatories to support the health of clergy and religious leaders. In addition to leading or speaking at conferences on clergy health, I've enjoyed writing a blog twice a week that mostly focuses on clergy health from various perspectives www.smccutchan.com. I've written several books that address particular aspects of clergy well-being. They are all available on Amazon, and you can read about them on my Website www.smccutchan.com I would particularly call your attention to the Healthy Clergy Make Healthy Congregations series. (HCMHC)

I've written devotional reflections on each passage of the lectionary that might contribute to your continuing spiritual journey. And, if you enjoy fictional stories that involve clergy, there are a couple of novels as well.

Now I am drawing upon ten years of writing and speaking to create six small books under the theme of **Healthy Clergy Make Healthy Congregations.** This first book addresses the issue of physical health. Future volumes in the series will look at emotional, family, financial, spiritual, and vocational health. I have deliberately kept them inexpensive so that clergy, congregations, and judicatories can afford to make them available to those who would benefit from them. Each will be available in both electronic and print form.

I believe in the clergy. I recognize that ordination does not protect clergy from the same type of human foibles that plague the rest of humanity. In some ways, the ministry can confront them with even more temptations. Recall that Jesus experienced his most direct temptations upon receiving God's call and affirmation at baptism.

Scripture teaches me that God is quite capable of calling imperfect people through which God can communicate the hope of the Gospel. I want to provide strategies and insight that can assist these servants of the Lord to be vehicles of God's grace. By offering ways to address the challenges to their health, I hope to support them in being trusting servants that can guide our churches in being faithful. amzn.to/13VO446

RESOURCES BY STEPHEN McCUTCHAN

HEALTHY CLERGY MAKE HEALTHY CONGREGATIONS

A Company of Pastors   bit.ly/CompanyofPastors

An Interim Pastor's Gift   bit.ly/InterimGift

God Laughs—Why Don't You?   bit.ly/Godlaughs

Clergy Physical Health

  http://bit.ly/clergyphyshealth

Clergy Emotional Health

Clergy Family Health

Clergy Financial Health

Clergy Spiritual Health

Clergy Vocational Health

FICTION

Clergy Tales—Tails (3 Volumes)

   bit.ly/3volClergyTales

A Star & A Tear (a mystery novel)   amzn.to/1aTDdgs

Blessed Are the Peacemakers http://bit.ly/BlessPeace

(A psychological thriller)

(All available on Amazon or www.smccutchan.com)

THE WATER SERIES

(A CSS Pub devotional series based on the Revised

Common Lectionary)   www.csspub.com

Water From the Well   (Year A)

Streams of Living Water   (Year B)

Water From the Rock   (Year C)

BIBLICAL RESOURCES

Experiencing the Psalms   www.helwys.com

Good News for a Fractured Society

http://bit.ly/GNFractSoc

CDS DESIGNED FOR SUPPORT OF PASTORS

A Deep Well for the Pastor

Laughter From the Well

www.smccutchan.com

COMMUNITY ISSUES

Let's Have Lunch

amzn.to/12ErVoL

Conversation, Race, and Community

ABOUT THE AUTHOR

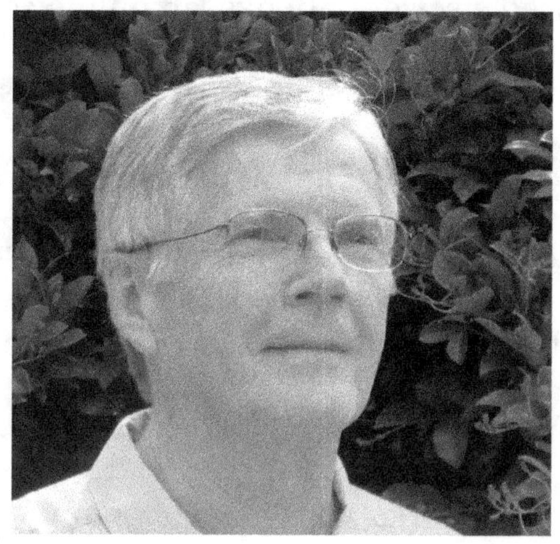

Stephen McCutchan

www.smccutchan.com

A PASTOR WHO LOVES THE

CHURCH

I am an ordained Presbyterian minister. After thirty-eight

years serving the church as a pastor, in retirement I have

focused my energies on developing resources in support of the clergy who continue to serve the church.

As a writer, humorist, and advocate for the care of clergy, I have authored a series of books, an online course on Matthew and two CDs in support of various aspects of ministry by clergy. Now I am writing a series, *Healthy Clergy Make Healthy Congregations*. (HCMHC). Nine volumes will address a broad range of issues affecting the health of clergy and other religious leaders

All my published works are available on my Website *www.smccutchan.com* as well as my weekly blog on various practical ways that clergy, congregations, and denominations can practice healthy ministry.

My hope is that each of these volumes will be helpful in the support of healthy clergy and healthy churches. If you have read this far, I know that you share this concern. We all believe that healthier churches contribute to the well being of our society.

If these books provide valuable insight in achieving the goal of healthy clergy, then I ask you to do four things.

➢ **Tell clergy, churches, and judicatories about these resources.**

➢ **Implement some of the strategies on behalf of yourself and other clergy.**

➢ **Write reviews on Amazon about these books.**

➢ **Be intentional about managing your own health.**